EFFORTLESS BODY DETOX

Renew Your Vitality And

Wellness With Ease

KARRY WILSON

ISBN: 9798861722087

Contents

INTRODUCTION

Our bodies are subjected to a constant barrage of toxins and pollutants. From the air we breathe to the food we consume, harmful substances can accumulate, leaving us feeling sluggish, fatigued, and far from our best selves. But what if there was a straightforward, painless way to hit the reset button on your health and vitality?

You will discover the power of gentle and effective detoxification to rejuvenate your body, mind, and spirit. This isn't about extreme diets, grueling cleanses, or unattainable wellness goals. Instead, it's a holistic approach to wellness that is both achievable and sustainable.

We'll embark on a journey to understand the science behind detoxification, explore the benefits it offers, and equip you with practical, everyday strategies to seamlessly integrate detox principles into your life. Whether you're a detox novice or someone looking to refine your approach, this guide is designed to meet you where you are on your wellness path.

By the time you turn the final page, you'll have the knowledge, tools, and inspiration to make effortless body detox a lifelong habit, one that renews your vitality, boosts your immunity, and restores your overall sense of well-being. So, let's embark on this transformative journey together, where you'll find that detoxifying your body can be as simple as it is rewarding.

CHAPTER 1

The Art of Body Detox

Are you yearning for a comprehensive body makeover? If so, step into the world of body detox, where you can embark on a 10-day journey to rejuvenate your entire being. This isn't just a cleanse; it's a holistic transformation that encompasses dietary changes, exercise, and much more.

A full-body detox goes beyond the short-term fixes of a 24-hour fast or a 72-hour juice diet. It's a program that requires your dedication and time to unlock its full potential. You'll need a system that:

Rids your body of heavy metals like lead and mercury.

Detoxifies vital organs, including the liver, kidneys, and even the brain.

Replenishes beneficial bacteria with a powerful probiotic formula.

Boosts your immune system with potent antioxidant support.

But detoxing isn't just about the physical; it's also about revitalizing your mind and spirit. Your brain deserves a detox too, although it's a different kind of cleansing.

While your brain benefits from the detox of your body's organs, cleansing your soul requires a unique approach. To truly refresh and rejuvenate your entire being during a 10-day full-body detox, take time to relax, recharge, and retrain your mind.

It's an opportunity to unwind from the daily worries and troubles, aligning your mental and spiritual well-being with your physical detox.

Consider incorporating journaling, mindfulness exercises, and deep breathing into your regimen alongside dietary changes. By the end of this process, you'll emerge as a renewed and reinvigorated version of yourself.

Understanding the Essence of a Body Detox Routine

Planning a body detox to revitalize your health? Whether you're a newbie or a seasoned detox enthusiast, having a well-structured detox routine is crucial. So, what exactly does a detox routine entail?

In essence, a detox routine is a natural approach to cleansing your body, providing it with the time and conditions needed to repair and recover from the daily wear and tear, as well as the effects of your dietary and lifestyle choices.

There's a multitude of detox routines to choose from, each with its own unique approach. Some popular options include:

Juice fasting

Herbal detoxification

Water fasting

Caloric restriction

Minimal eating/fasting

Herbal detoxification

Detox baths

Colon cleansing

And many more

Your detox routine is the specific plan you adopt to detoxify and rejuvenate your body. It could be a pre-designed program that provides all the necessary steps for a healthy detox, or it might be a routine you've customized to suit your preferences.

Feel free to experiment with different detox routines or combinations thereof until you discover the one that resonates best with you.

Once you find your ideal routine, you can return to it whenever your body calls for a detox.

The frequency of your detox sessions depends on your chosen routine, your lifestyle, and your commitment to maintaining a healthy diet and lifestyle afterward.

If you continue to eat healthily and avoid toxin-rich substances post-detox, you won't need to detox as frequently.

However, if you revert to an unhealthy diet, caffeine, sugar, or nicotine, you'll accumulate toxins faster, necessitating more frequent detox sessions.

Remember, your detox routine is a tailored approach to reclaiming your vitality and well-being, and its frequency should align with your unique journey to a healthier you.

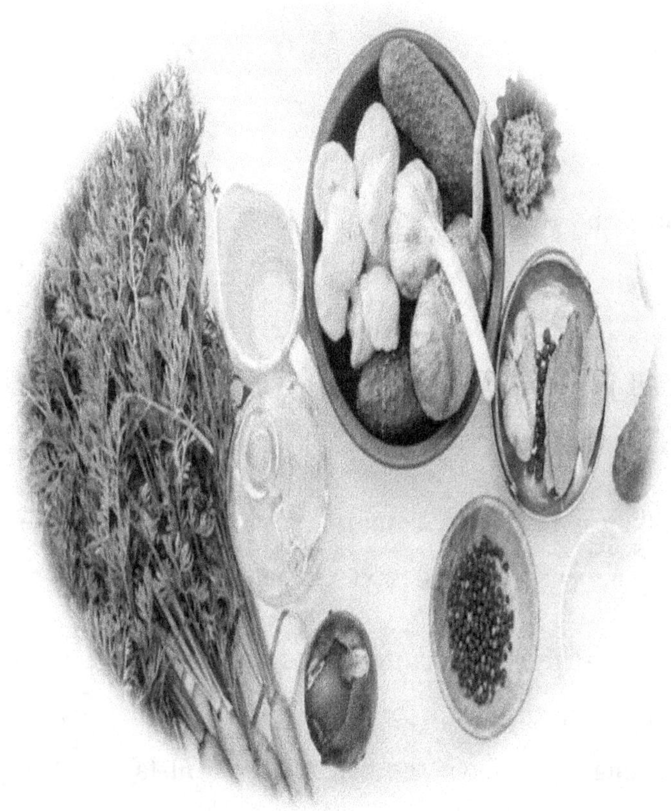

CHAPTER 2

The Power of Keeping a Body Detox Journal

Embarking on a body detox journey? Here's a modern twist that can make a world of difference: keeping a detox journal. Forget the traditional notebook; you can choose a digital journaling app or even a voice recording device if that's more your style.

The key is to have a comfortable and convenient method for documenting your detox experience.

Your journal can be as unique as you are. The purpose is simple: record your life and experiences during the detox. You might jot down the detox steps you take, what you consume, what you restrict, and any reactions your body exhibits.

However, don't stop there. Embrace the freedom to document your feelings and emotions throughout this journey.

Even if they don't seem directly related to your detox, they can provide valuable insights when you reflect on your experience later.

Benefits of Maintaining a Body Detox Journal

The advantages of keeping a detox journal are manifold. Firstly, it acts as a personal guide for your detox journey.

By noting the steps you take and your experiences, you create a valuable reference for future detoxes.

If something didn't work well for you, your journal will be your guide to make adjustments next time. Over the years, you can compare your detox experiences, track changes, and witness your personal growth.

Moreover, detoxification often triggers mood swings and emotional turbulence. Your journal becomes your emotional compass, helping you navigate these feelings. It's a tool for self-reflection and emotional growth.

Reading through your past entries, you can observe how you've evolved emotionally, gaining valuable insights into your own psyche.

Detox Your Mind

While body detox gets its fair share of attention, detoxifying your mind is equally vital. Stress, worries, and fears are constant companions in our daily lives, and they can accumulate, cluttering our mental space. To declutter your mind, consider establishing regular "cleansing days," not as a one-time event but as an ongoing practice.

Start with a journaling habit. Write daily about your feelings, experiences, and thoughts. If daily journaling feels overwhelming, designate a specific day, perhaps once a week or every two weeks, for your mental detox.

Express yourself in letters, even if you never intend to send them. These letters can serve as a safe outlet for your emotions, helping you release the stress that accumulates in your mind.

Remember, the goal isn't to suppress negative emotions. Instead, acknowledge and embrace them. Use them as stepping stones to personal growth. Holding onto past pains and regrets only allows them to fester, ultimately harming your mental well-being.

These steps toward mental detoxification can lead to a fresher, more positive outlook on life. Clearing your mental clutter will not only improve your emotional well-being but also contribute to your overall health and vitality.

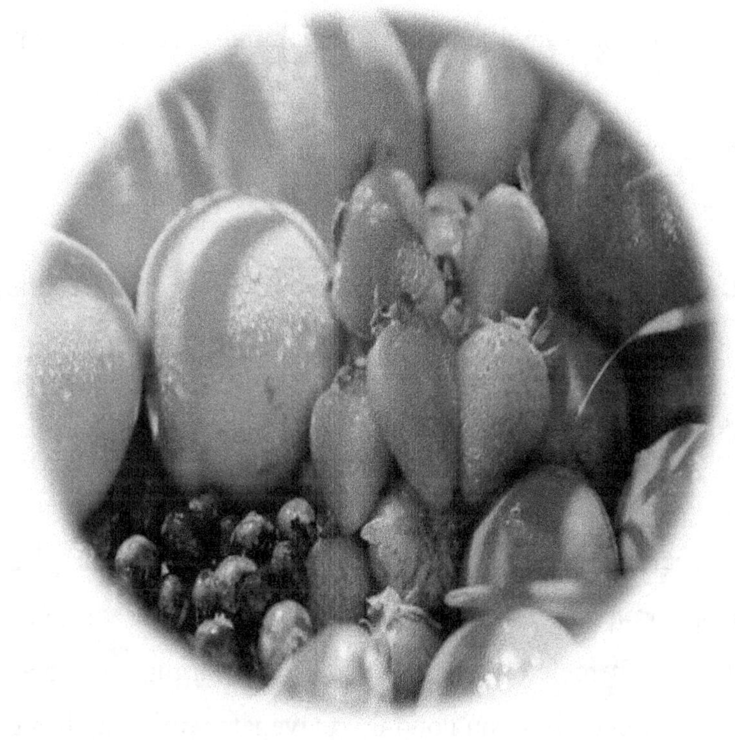

CHAPTER 3

Reveal Your Best Skin Through Body Detox

Body detox isn't just about internal health; it can work wonders for your skin too. While you might be aware of its benefits in cleansing your colon, eliminating toxins, and boosting your overall health, you might not know that it's also a secret weapon for achieving fantastic skin.

If you're yearning for youthful, smooth, and radiant skin, detoxifying your body might be the path to follow.

A Mirror of Inner Health

Your skin often reflects your internal well-being. Unhealthy individuals tend to have dry, lackluster skin, more pronounced wrinkles, and premature signs of aging. This is where detoxification steps in. By purging your body of harmful toxins, you not only rejuvenate your inner health but also reveal a refreshed, glowing complexion.

Toxins accumulate within your body over time, causing your skin to appear dull and lifeless. They can also accelerate the aging process, contributing to the early onset of fine lines and wrinkles.

Deep detoxification from the inside-out removes these burdens from your body and revitalizes your skin. In the days following your detox, you'll likely notice your skin becoming healthier and more vibrant.

Sustaining the Glow

To maintain your newfound radiance, consider making hydration a priority. Drinking ample water, whether prescribed in your detox program or not, can be exceptionally beneficial. Proper hydration ensures that your skin remains supple and well-nourished.

If you have specific skin concerns like acne or other dermatological issues, there are specialized skin detox formulas available. These are tailored to address problem skin conditions or signs of aging, such as fine lines and wrinkles.

By incorporating these targeted detox systems, you can rejuvenate your skin and achieve a more youthful appearance.

Remember, your skin is not just a superficial layer; it's a reflection of your inner health. A body detox not only revitalizes your body but also helps you put your best face forward, quite literally. So, as you embark on this journey, anticipate not only a healthier internal you but also a more radiant, confident exterior.

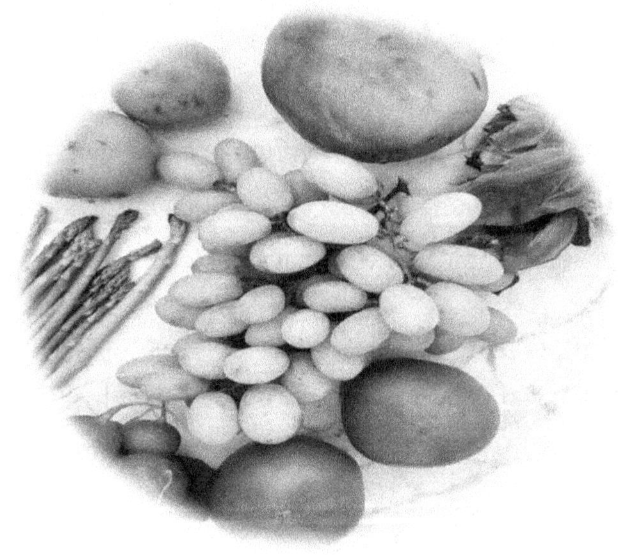

CHAPTER 4

Simplifying Your Self-Detox Journey

In today's world, achieving a 100 percent toxin-free existence within our bodies is an elusive goal.

Detoxification isn't always a seamless process, and sometimes, our bodies need a helping hand to effectively rid themselves of accumulated toxins.

Fortunately, there are various methods to assist in this natural cleansing process, including dietary changes, detox kits, and herbal detoxification tonics and pills.

It's essential to debunk the myth that we are toxin-free just because we maintain a clean lifestyle. The reality is quite different. Toxins infiltrate our bodies through various avenues. Pesticides linger on the vegetables we consume, even after thorough washing.

Air pollution, laden with smoke and petroleum fumes, continuously exposes us to toxins. Additionally, everyday household products like toiletries and cleaning agents contain chemicals that infiltrate our bodies through the skin, eyes, and respiratory system, accumulating over time.

These toxins, if not adequately flushed from our systems, can lead to health problems. Consequently, periodic detoxification is crucial to prevent a dangerous buildup of toxins in the body.

While modern medicine has made significant strides in extending human life and alleviating disease symptoms, it's essential to acknowledge that many medications leave behind residue that transforms into toxins within our bodies. Even seemingly innocuous drugs contribute to toxin accumulation. It's imperative to expel these toxins to maintain good health.

Our kidneys and liver play a significant role in detoxifying our bodies, but when toxin levels become overwhelming, we need external assistance. Here's where detox kits come into play. These kits typically contain herbal detox products that complement a specified dietary plan. When used correctly, they can effectively eliminate toxins from the body in as little as five days.

However, finding the right detox product for your needs may require some trial and error. Each person's body is unique, and what works for one might not work for another. But with some patience and experimentation, you will eventually discover the ideal detox product that aligns with your body's requirements.

Detoxification isn't a one-time process but a lifestyle choice. Regular detox routines, tailored to your unique needs, can help you maintain optimal health, bolster your immune system, and ensure you're free from the burden of accumulated toxins.

In the next chapters, we will explore various detox methods, dietary changes, and lifestyle adjustments to assist you on your journey towards a healthier, toxin-free you.

CHAPTER 5

The Science of Internal Cleansing: Detoxifying Your Body

The battle against toxins is constant. Each day, our bodies encounter an onslaught of pollutants and chemicals from various sources.

These insidious toxins can wreak havoc on our vital organs, leaving destruction in their wake. But fear not, for there are ways to cleanse your body from the inside out, rejuvenating your health and vitality.

Understanding Toxins

Toxins come at us from every angle. The very air we breathe carries a payload of pollutants from car exhaust and industrial emissions. Even the seemingly innocent act of eating our daily greens can expose us to toxins through the pesticides and chemical fertilizers used in farming. The water we drink is often treated with chemicals for purification, and these chemicals inevitably find their way into our bodies.

Medications, intended to heal, often leave a residue of toxins within our system. Even personal care products, such as deodorants and sprays, can contribute to our toxic burden.

The Impact of Toxins

Toxins take a toll on our organs, primarily targeting the kidneys, liver, and colon. They can compromise our immune system, making our bodies susceptible to diseases and deteriorating our overall health.

Some common symptoms of toxin overload include premature aging, skin issues like rashes, indigestion, nausea, and behavioral changes, including depression.

The Detox Solution

To combat this constant assault of toxins, it's essential to embark on a detoxification journey. One effective approach is the detox diet.

This regimen centers around consuming an abundance of vegetables and fruits, ideally for a five-day period, complemented by a daily intake of at least 4 liters of water. This strategy alone can eliminate over 80% of toxins from your system.

Alternatively, there are home detox kits available that include herbal detox pills and tonics. These kits work in tandem with your organs to systematically detoxify your body.

Regardless of the method you choose, regular detoxification is key, with a recommended frequency of twice a year. A detoxified body is not only a healthier one but also a happier one.

In the upcoming chapters, we will delve deeper into various detox approaches, helping you achieve a cleaner, more vibrant you.

CHAPTER 6

The Herbal Revolution: Detox Your Life with Nature's Bounty

Our environment and dietary choices bombard us with a barrage of harmful chemicals that silently infiltrate our bodies.

Pesticides, air pollutants, and a myriad of artificial additives find their way into our systems, accumulating over time to wreak havoc on our well-being. This relentless buildup of toxins necessitates a powerful cleansing process, aptly named detoxification.

While our bodies possess natural detoxification mechanisms, these vital systems can become overwhelmed by the onslaught of modern-day toxins. That's when they need a little help from us to restore balance to our circulatory and excretory systems. While some resort to unhealthy practices like prolonged fasting, a more sensible approach is to adopt a detox diet, complemented by the remarkable power of detoxifying herbs.

The Consequences of Toxin Accumulation

Toxins gradually weaken our immune system, leaving us susceptible to various illnesses. It's crucial to remove these harmful substances through a detox process to maintain a robust defense against disease.

The medical community recognizes the potent detoxifying abilities of herbs, which offer a natural and effective solution for cleansing the body and nurturing a sense of overall well-being.

Harnessing Nature's Detoxifying Herbs

Several herbs stand out for their exceptional detoxifying properties:

Psyllium Seeds: These seeds act as effective bowel movers, cleansing the intestines of toxins. They function like sponges, absorbing harmful substances and eliminating them through excretion.

Cascara Sagrada: Another potent laxative, cascara sagrada, is often used alongside psyllium seeds to flush toxins from the system.

Milk Thistle: Known to stimulate protein synthesis in the liver, the body's primary blood-cleansing organ, milk thistle supports detoxification.

Nettles: Used in conjunction with other detox herbs, nettles help purify the urinary system, eliminating toxins.

Burdock Roots: When immediate detoxification is essential, burdock roots come into play. These herbs reduce the accumulation of metals in the body, a common source of health problems.

Dandelion Roots: Boasting the most robust detoxifying properties, dandelion roots are instrumental in cleansing the gall bladder and kidneys. They are often used in combination with other detox herbs to ensure a comprehensive detoxification process.

The primary sources of toxins for humans are air pollution and the toxins present in processed foods. Due to time constraints, people are increasingly turning to processed foods, often unaware of the health risks they entail. Detoxification, therefore, becomes a necessary ritual for many, undertaken at least twice a year.

Medical experts concur that detoxifying the system is vital, emphasizing that a more natural approach is not only better but also safer for our long-term well-being.

In the chapters ahead, we'll delve deeper into specific detoxification strategies, guiding you toward a healthier and revitalized you.

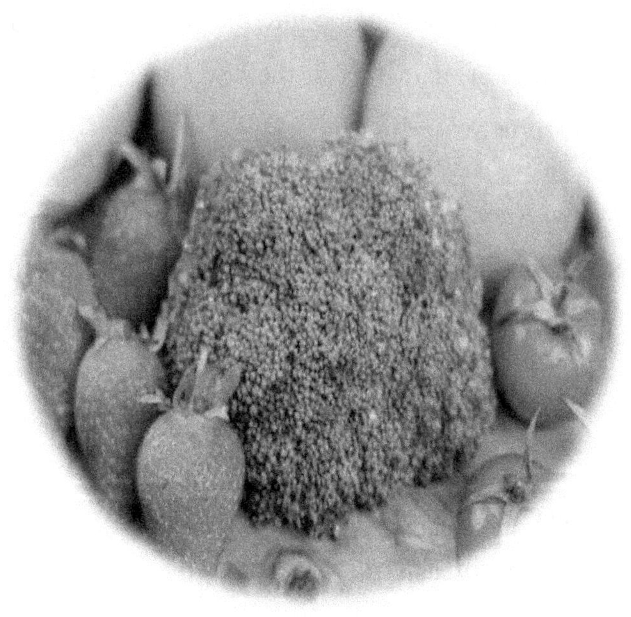

CHAPTER 7

Fueling Your Vitality: The Art of Nutritional Detox

Signs of sluggishness, perpetual fullness, indigestion, or persistent feelings of excess weight can often be attributed to a buildup of toxins in the body. Sometimes, our bodies send out clear signals that it's time to detoxify.

These signals might manifest as an aversion to rich or overly sweet foods, even causing slight nausea at their sight. These are signs that your liver might be struggling with an excessive toxic load, and it's high time to pay attention and take action.

Understanding Detoxification

Detoxification is a systematic approach to reducing or eliminating harmful toxins from the body. Many detox plans are available for those seeking to cleanse their systems. While detox massages, medications, and yoga can play a role, the cornerstone of detoxification is a well-structured detox diet plan.

The Power of a Detox Diet

A detox diet plan is your roadmap to not only what to eat but also when and how to eat for a healthier you. It's an educational journey that helps you understand the value of proper nutrition, leading to a potentially toxin-free life.

Natural Food as Your Ally

The core of a detox diet is organic, natural foods, primarily consisting of green leafy vegetables and fruits.

These unprocessed, preservative-free ingredients are readily absorbed by your body, eliminating the need to work tirelessly to expel harmful chemicals often found in processed foods.

Natural foods are rich in antioxidants, vitamins, and minerals crucial for nurturing a healthy body and mind. Additionally, they provide essential dietary fibers necessary for tissue repair.

A Word of Caution

While detox diets offer numerous benefits, they may not be suitable for everyone. If you are pregnant or planning to become pregnant, it's advisable to stick to your regular diet until after delivery, as your body requires extra energy during this period.

A sudden shift to a detox diet may not be conducive to your well-being or that of your baby.

Furthermore, remember that balance is key. Excessive detoxification can be detrimental, so it's wise to consult with your healthcare provider before embarking on a detox plan.

Incorporating a detox diet into your life can yield significant advantages, and it's a practice that should be considered at least once a year. By learning to nourish your body with the right foods, you'll not only experience the rejuvenating effects of detoxification but also lay the foundation for a long-lasting, healthy lifestyle.

CHAPTER 8

The Pursuit of Wellness: Holistic Detox for Body and Mind

The term 'toxin' often conjures images of poison bottles marked with skull and crossbones. But not all toxins come with warning labels; many silently infiltrate our bodies through the food and drinks we consume, as well as the air we breathe and the water we drink.

These toxins aren't visible to the naked eye, but their cumulative impact can be profound, affecting our biological systems over time.

Invisible Intruders

Toxins can be microscopic bacteria or pollutants used in food processing and preservation. They infiltrate our bodies over the years, often unnoticed, causing havoc within our biological systems. Additionally, toxins permeate our environment, present in the air we breathe and the water we drink. They even penetrate our skin through pores and enter our lungs with every breath. It's imperative to eliminate these pollutants from our systems before they compromise our health and well-being.

Regular detoxification is the answer, and it can be achieved through a well-structured detox diet.

Why Can't Our Bodies Do It Alone?

One might wonder, "Why can't our bodies naturally eliminate the toxins we encounter?" The answer is simple. While our bodies have a built-in detoxification system, it has its limits.

As pollution levels have surged to unprecedented heights, our bodies struggle to keep up. This is precisely why we need to make wise dietary choices and engage in regular detox routines.

Traditional Wisdom: A Lesson for Modern Life

In days past, our parents would often administer purgatives to periodically cleanse our systems of toxins. They also emphasized the importance of drinking pure water, a practice worth passing down to future generations. Opting for whole, healthy foods over today's processed alternatives is a choice we should embrace to nourish our bodies.

Ditch the Junk, Embrace the Natural

The safest way to detoxify our bodies is through a natural process. This begins by bidding farewell to junk food, notorious for its preservatives, excess oil, and grease content. Fast food, as it's often called, should be a rarity in our diets.

Certain products like alcohol, fats, and caffeine contribute significantly to toxin levels within the body. To combat this, shift towards a diet rich in fiber from fruits and vegetables. This natural diet facilitates the gentle expulsion of toxins without the need for medications.

It's prudent to limit meat consumption and alcohol intake, reserving them for occasional treats. By adhering primarily to a diet centered around fruits and vegetables, we can proactively keep toxins at bay and embrace a healthier, toxin-free life.

CHAPTER 9

The Safe Path to Detox: Navigating Your Body's Cleansing Journey

In the hustle and bustle of our daily lives, we are constantly exposed to a multitude of toxins lurking in the atmosphere. The water we drink, once thought to be pure, now raises concerns about its purity.

To top it off, our modern diets are often laden with preservatives and processed foods that contribute to the toxic cocktail swirling within our bodies.

The Silent Accumulators: Toxins

Toxins aren't just an abstract concept; they actively harm our well-being. Removing these insidious intruders from our system is essential. This task falls upon the shoulders of a well-structured detox regime, typically spanning anywhere from a brief 5 days to a more comprehensive 2 weeks. Central to this regimen is the detox diet, a diet that thrives on the essence of nature.

It means embracing foods untouched by processing, or at the very least, minimally processed and devoid of added preservatives.

A typical detox diet revolves around fresh fruits and vegetables, prepared with minimal or no oils and fats.

These unadulterated foods are your allies in purging your body of toxins, leading to a rejuvenated and healthier self. Throughout this process, adequate hydration is paramount, and you should aim to consume at least three liters of water each day.

From Celebrities to Everyday Heroes: The Detox Movement

Detox diets have garnered attention not only from celebrities but also from individuals looking to break free from the clutches of excessive alcohol consumption or simply cleanse their bodies of accumulated toxins. But the question that often arises is, "Are detox diets safe?" The safety of detox diets hinges on a crucial factor: control. Unsupervised detox diets can lead to adverse effects. A prudent approach is to adhere to a diet primarily composed of fruits and lightly cooked vegetables, paired with ample water intake, for a minimum of 8 days.

This sensible strategy will effectively cleanse your system of harmful toxins while preserving your well-being.

The Body's Natural Cleansing Mechanism

The human body has a built-in mechanism to eliminate toxins. Organs like the kidneys, liver, and intestines tirelessly work to process the food and drink we consume, expelling toxins through urine, excreta, and sweat.

However, this process is efficient only up to a certain toxin threshold. When toxin levels soar beyond this threshold, the body requires our intervention to maintain a healthy equilibrium.

Remember the fundamental lessons from your school days: chew your food thoroughly before swallowing. It's not just a childhood mantra; it's a healthy habit. In fact, there's wisdom in chewing each bite at least 32 times, as it aids digestion. A wholesome diet plan might include brown bread, modest servings of rice, and generous portions of fiber-rich foods. Reducing sugar and spices while upping your water intake can significantly enhance your overall health and vitality.

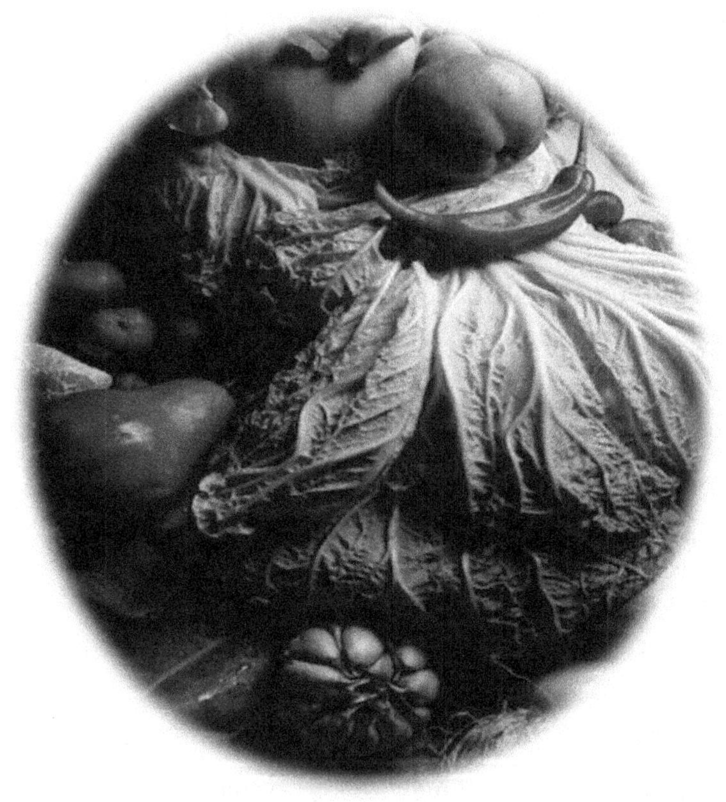

CHAPTER 10

Unleash a Fresher You with a 5-Day Detox Journey

In our modern era, escaping the clutches of pollutants that silently infiltrate our system is nigh impossible. Pollution is omnipresent, weaving itself into the fabric of our daily lives.

It lurks at work, haunts public spaces, taints the food we consume, and even tinges the water we rely on for sustenance.

Picture this: a chance encounter with a nonchalant smoker in a public place, indifferent to the plumes of smoke drifting your way.

Or perhaps the olfactory assault of perfumes and restroom sprays that you involuntarily inhale, further contributing to the burgeoning toxin load within your body.

So, how can we tackle this menace of toxins, and what havoc do they wreak in the first place?

The Toxic Toll: Unmasking the Intruders

Toxins, insidious as they are, inflict an array of harm upon our bodies. They accelerate the aging process, leading to unsightly wrinkles and pave the way for various illnesses and conditions like skin irritations and digestive disturbances.

While the body boasts its own detoxification mechanisms, some toxins require a nudge from us.

The body, despite its resilience, cannot indefinitely cope with the ceaseless influx of toxins. It needs our support.

Proactive Detoxification: A Prescription for Vitality

Waiting for your body to raise a red flag, signaling the need for a detox, isn't wise.

The wisdom lies in regular, proactive detoxification. Ideally, you should undertake a detox every few months to maintain your health and preserve your harmonious relationships.

The Power of a 5-Day Detox Plan

When pollutants overwhelm your system, your tissues become strained, and your organs start to falter. This is when the clarion call for detoxification rings out. However, why wait for such dire circumstances? Embrace the 5-day detox plan as a preventative measure.

During this brief but potent detox journey, certain foods must be avoided. Focus on consuming fresh green vegetables and a bounty of fruits. It's crucial to steer clear of oils, fats, preservatives, and any foods laden with unnatural additives, as these culprits significantly contribute to the toxin overload.

The 5-day detox plan advocates for a complete halt to meat consumption. Instead, opt for a diet rich in vegetables and fruits, minus the oils.

You'll witness a tangible shift in your health as early as the 3rd day of this regimen, and the transformation is truly invigorating!

CHAPTER 11

Gentle Paths to a Cleaner You

Every day, toxins stealthily infiltrate our bodies, sneaking in through the food we consume, the beverages we savor, and the air we breathe.

Even our daily shower exposes us to these unwanted invaders, as they slip through our skin's pores.

They sap our vitality, leave us weary, and provoke bodily discomfort - unmistakable signals that our system cries out for detoxification.

Unleash Your Inner Radiance

If you seek a clearer, more vibrant complexion, heightened energy levels, a fortified immune system, and enhanced mental acuity, it's high time to consider detoxifying your body. This process primarily focuses on purifying your blood by expelling toxins. The key players in this purification symphony are the kidneys, liver, and the lymphatic system.

Charting Your Detox Course

Embarking on a detox journey requires some essential changes. Firstly, bid farewell to alcohol and cigarettes.

Additionally, you must steer clear of fats, processed foods, coffee, and fizzy drinks - all of which serve as toxin reservoirs and must be eliminated.

Then, let's tackle other overlooked culprits. Household cleaning agents and personal care products, like chemical-laden shampoos, deodorants, and toothpaste, often introduce toxins into our systems, wreaking havoc beneath the surface.

Now, with a myriad of detox methods available, the challenge is to choose the one that aligns with your preferences. Here are some approaches to consider:

Fasting: This age-old practice is the cornerstone of detoxification. Our ancestors fasted for system cleansing long before we knew the term "toxin."

Fasting remains a powerful way to purge the body of harmful substances.

Juice Power: Embrace a fruit and vegetable juice diet. Carrots, spinach, celery, cabbage, apples, and pineapple juices work wonders. Commit to this regimen for at least five days, and exclude citrus fruit juices.

Weight Loss Journey: Combine fasting with exercise. It's well-documented that obese individuals harbor the highest toxin levels. A 30-day juice fast can help shed at least 30 pounds of excess weight.

Weeklong Veggie Odyssey: Opt for a weeklong vegetarian diet rich in leafy greens and ample fruit. Hydrate yourself generously with at least 4 liters of water daily.

By diligently adhering to a well-tailored detox regimen, you'll effectively expel accumulated toxins, ushering in a healthier, more productive version of yourself.

CHAPTER 12

Harmonizing pH and Detox for a Cleaner You

Your body's pH levels play a crucial role in maintaining overall health. When your pH becomes overly acidic, it can lead to fatigue, weight gain, digestive issues, and various discomforts.

Prolonged acidity can even result in more severe health problems. In such cases, it's time to consider detoxification, a process that purges harmful toxins from your body and restores a natural alkaline pH balance.

While the body has a natural detoxification mechanism, it can sometimes be overwhelmed by an excess of harmful toxins.

This overload can occur during illness, when bodily functions are compromised, or when we neglect a healthy diet and lifestyle. Overconsumption of acidic foods further disrupts the balance, and a sedentary lifestyle hinders the body's ability to eliminate toxins.

Detoxification is a route to better health and enhanced productivity, regardless of how these imbalances occur.

The body's effort to maintain a healthy blood pH level is as diligent as its temperature regulation. Normally, our blood pH hovers slightly above 7, and our body makes considerable efforts to sustain this balance, even straining tissues and organs to do so.

Surprisingly, even within the standard pH range, an imbalance can lead to health issues.

As mentioned earlier, excessive fatigue, weight gain, digestion problems, and general discomfort might signal an out-of-balance pH level.

These symptoms often indicate an overload of acids in your system, whether through diet, internal production, or inefficient elimination.

A straightforward way to detoxify from excess acids is to revamp your diet. Acidic-contributing foods, such as dairy, processed sugars, red meat, alcohol, coffee, and carbonated beverages, should be minimized. Consuming excessive amounts of these items may overwhelm your body's natural acid-neutralizing capacity and hinder it from returning to a balanced alkaline state.

Acidifying toxins can also originate from microorganisms (microscopic animal or plant organisms) and pathogens within the body.

While every human body harbors microorganisms that assist in digestion, an overabundance of these microorganisms can lead to excessive acid production, impair digestion, and potentially result in conditions like irritable bowel syndrome, Crohn's disease, and even colon cancer.

These pathogens can enter the bloodstream, carrying diseases to cells, tissues, and entire biological systems. An out-of-balance pH level can be an indicator of such occurrences.

Detoxification is the solution, but an overwhelmed system can't manage it alone. You must intervene to restore a healthy pH balance. A detox diet should comprise highly alkaline foods like vegetables and low-sugar fruits, ample hydration through alkaline water, and appropriate alkaline-rich supplements.

Alkalizing products are available to help restore your pH balance. Tasteless, odorless structured alkaline waters are designed for optimal absorption and contain minerals that aid in achieving a healthy pH balance.

These waters neutralize acids and eliminate toxins. When using alkaline waters as part of a detox diet, aim to consume three to four liters (about 3-4 quarts) daily.

Dietary alkaline supplements contain essential minerals like calcium, magnesium, and iron, replenishing your body's mineral reserves and buffering acids.

Some of these mineral-rich supplements also promote the efficient elimination of acids from the body.

However, always consult your doctor before embarking on a detox diet or taking supplements to ensure proper diagnosis and treatment.

CHAPTER 13

Embrace a Clean and Detoxed Lifestyle for Optimal Well-being

Talk of detoxification is more pertinent than ever. Detox isn't reserved solely for recovery from substances like drugs or alcohol; it's a practice for everyone.

We exist in an environment riddled with air and water pollution, coupled with unhealthy habits. Chemicals, both beneficial and harmful, envelop us at every turn.

In today's fast-paced life, we inundate our bodies with processed foods, fast foods, and an array of preservatives and additives.

Additionally, the emergence of genetically modified "designer" foods adds another layer of uncertainty to their impact on our health.

Amid this dietary chaos, the silver lining is that people are becoming more conscious of what they eat.

When we discuss "detoxification," we're referring to the process of eliminating toxins from our bodies.

In this context, body detox employs diets, herbs, and other methods to remove toxins and promote improved health.

If you're concerned about your health and the toxins that may be accumulating in your body, it's time to explore the concept of body detox.

It's a health-conscious choice in an increasingly unhealthy world. However, keep in mind that body detox necessitates a lifestyle shift.

This shift involves adopting a more balanced diet consisting of natural, wholesome foods, increased water intake, and regular physical activity.

It means steering clear of fast food, processed meals (including frozen dinners and canned goods), and other dietary culprits.

While this transformation may not be instantaneous, you can start today by changing your approach to food.

A revamped lifestyle also translates to incorporating more regular exercise into your routine. You don't need a gym membership or fancy workout attire; simply move more.

Go for brisk walks, choose stairs over elevators, and carry your groceries to the car. There are countless ways to increase your physical activity without even realizing it.

For those serious about detoxing, a detox diet could be an option. It aims to reduce toxins in your body, alleviate aches and pains, ease allergies, enhance digestion, and boost energy levels.

Online resources offer numerous body detox recipes. Alternatively, visiting a local health food store can provide valuable insights into detoxifying foods and recipes.

A commitment to body detox means consuming abundant fresh fruits and prioritizing nuts, beans, rice, and whole grains over fried and gravy-laden dishes.

It also involves avoiding sugary desserts, caffeine, alcohol, yeast-rich foods, and processed products laden with questionable additives and preservatives.

If you're transitioning into or out of a body detox regimen, consider a one- or two-day fast. During your fast, ensure you stay well-hydrated, particularly with water.

Don't push yourself too hard; if hunger becomes overwhelming, opt for a piece of fruit or some carrot or celery sticks. Remember, you don't have to punish yourself during the detox process.

There are myriad other ways to detoxify and embrace a healthier lifestyle. Reconnect with nature by spending time outdoors.

Take leisurely walks at the beach, in your local park, or within a nature reserve. Prioritize "me time" within your daily schedule and make it a family affair as well.

Stay active and engaged with the world around you, get involved in community activities, and volunteer your time.

For a luxurious body detox experience, treat yourself to a spa day. Enjoy a relaxing massage or indulge in a deep-cleansing facial.

When showering, use a brush to expedite the detox process by gently enhancing circulation and shedding layers of toxin-laden dead skin.

Aid your body's natural toxin elimination process by drinking at least four quarts (about four liters) of water daily.

Consume fiber-rich foods like raspberries, blackberries, broccoli, apples (with the skin), spinach, almonds, peanuts, and whole wheat.

Additionally, explore teas and herbal supplements from your health food store that promote regular bowel movements.

Detoxifying the body involves a mental detox as well. Negative thinking can surprisingly contribute to toxin production and excessive acidity in the body. Rid yourself of worry, anger, and pessimism; they serve no positive purpose and are detrimental to your health. Smile until you genuinely feel like smiling.

The beauty of embarking on a body detox journey is that there's never a wrong time to start. In today's frantic, high-stress world, self-care is a necessity. Moreover, your family deserves the same healthy lifestyle.

Body detox can be as simple as altering your attitude, shedding negative, harmful thoughts that compromise your health. It can be as effortless as strolling in the park or indulging in a long, hot shower.

Alternatively, it can be as intricate as adopting and adhering to a stringent detox diet that cleanses your tissues and organs of harmful pathogens and excessive acidity.

The choice is yours, but the essence remains the same: embark on a journey to cleanse yourself.

Regardless of the path you choose, you're doing yourself and those around you a great service. You're reintroducing sanity into your life and setting an example for your children and social circle.

You're living better and savoring life more. This miraculous transformation doesn't require payment; it simply requires a change in your daily approach.

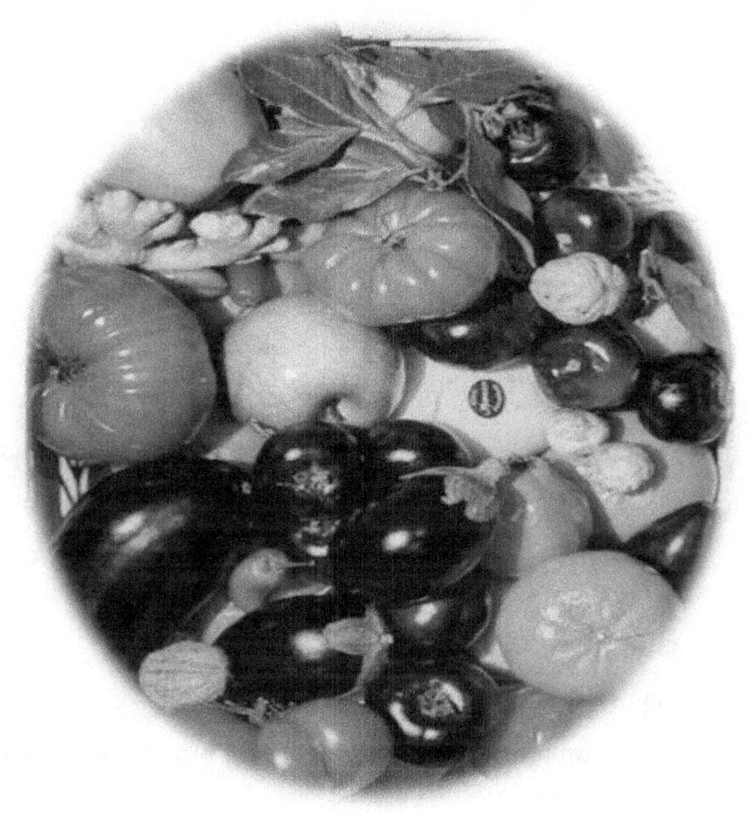

CHAPTER 14

Elevating Your Well-being through Body Detox: A Journey to Purify Body, Mind, and Soul

In the relentless hustle of the modern world, it's crucial to detoxify the human body. Detoxification, or detox for short, is about ridding the body of toxins and pathogens that accumulate over time, all in the pursuit of health and happiness.

The human body naturally expels toxins through biological processes and waste elimination. However, our contemporary environment relentlessly bombards us with pollutants, compromising our health and immune systems.

Body detox is a proactive approach where we consciously modify our dietary and lifestyle choices to enable the body to process and reduce toxins and pathogens to safe levels.

The primary culprit behind toxin buildup is an unhealthy diet. Fast food, junk food, and the preservatives and additives found in processed foods wreak havoc on our bodily functions.

Some of the most detrimental foods are those high in acidity, including caffeine, carbonated beverages, meat, sugary foods, and processed items (like canned and frozen foods).

A disrupted toxin balance can also result from bodily processes that aren't functioning optimally, particularly when waste elimination is hindered.

Participating in a well-structured body detox program can aid in restoring normal bodily functions.

When toxins surpass healthy levels within the body, it can manifest in symptoms such as fatigue, weight gain, muscle and joint pain, and, in severe cases, even cancer.

Scientists propose that an excessive production of free radicals initiates a chain reaction that overwhelms a healthy body. An overly acidic pH level in the body can contribute to these symptoms.

Health is a holistic concept encompassing not only physical well-being but also the intricate interactions of chemicals, hormones, and enzymes within our bodies that influence our emotions and thoughts.

Think back to your last illness – you likely remember feeling more negative and experiencing heightened emotional turmoil.

When our bodies are unhealthy, we tend to generate pessimistic thoughts and experience more destructive emotions. As physical stress increases, so does emotional stress.

Conversely, negative thoughts and destructive emotions can impact our health, weakening our immune systems and making us more susceptible to disease.

Body detox doesn't just cleanse our blood and organs; it purifies our minds and spirits, leading to improved overall health and well-being.

Detoxification, or detox, operates on multiple levels. Physically, it involves eliminating harmful substances from the body to restore a natural balance.

Remarkably, maintaining a healthy pH balance in the body is as crucial as maintaining an appropriate body temperature.

There's a plethora of body detox diets and programs available to guide you toward improved health. A simple internet search for "detox diet" or "body detox" will reveal a wealth of self-cleansing options. You can also seek advice from your local health food store.

Detoxification of the mind plays a significant role in a body detox program.

Reducing stress, worry, frustration, and anger in your daily life can expedite the detox process, assisting in the maintenance of healthy bodily functions and chemical balances.

By addressing your psychological and emotional needs, you can convert stress into joy and transform illness into robust health.

Eastern philosophers and religious leaders have long recognized the interconnectedness of physical well-being and spiritual harmony.

Fasting, a fundamental aspect of body detox, has historically aided in removing toxins from the body, resulting in mental clarity and emotional stability.

Although they may not have used the term "body detox," it's an inherent part of a healthy spiritual life.

Many professionals dedicated to physical, mental, and emotional healing contend that detoxification is essential in today's world.

A comprehensive body detox program, encompassing a healthier diet, regular exercise, and mindfulness of mental and emotional states, may be among the most positive changes we can make in our lives today.

Modern society is marked by pollution, stress, conflict, and confusion, factors beyond an individual's control. Yet, as individuals, we have the power to effect change, one person at a time, by adopting healthier, more positive lifestyles and outlooks.

Body detox does more than relieve physical discomfort or aid in weight loss; it transforms your life and your perspective on life itself.

You don't need to embark on a complex, formal body detox program to enhance your health. Small lifestyle changes can go a long way in revitalizing your health and perspective. Consider the following:

Drink 3-4 quarts of water daily.

Consume more vegetables and fruits and reduce meat and dairy intake.

Increase your regular physical exercise.

Experiment with short fasts lasting 1-2 days.

Limit or eliminate caffeine, sugary desserts, carbonated beverages, alcohol, milk chocolate, and high-acid foods.

Explore available alkalizing water and food supplements to restore a healthy pH balance.

Incorporate daily "me time" to regain mental and emotional equilibrium.

Delve into meditation or yoga practices.

A final piece of advice: before undertaking a detox diet or making significant changes to your diet or lifestyle, consult your healthcare provider. Ensure there are no underlying medical conditions requiring medical treatment before committing to a formal detox program.

Having said that, contemplate body detox as a means to enhance not only your life but also the lives of your loved ones. In a world filled with pollution and stress, making healthy, positive changes in our lifestyles is a step toward a brighter future.

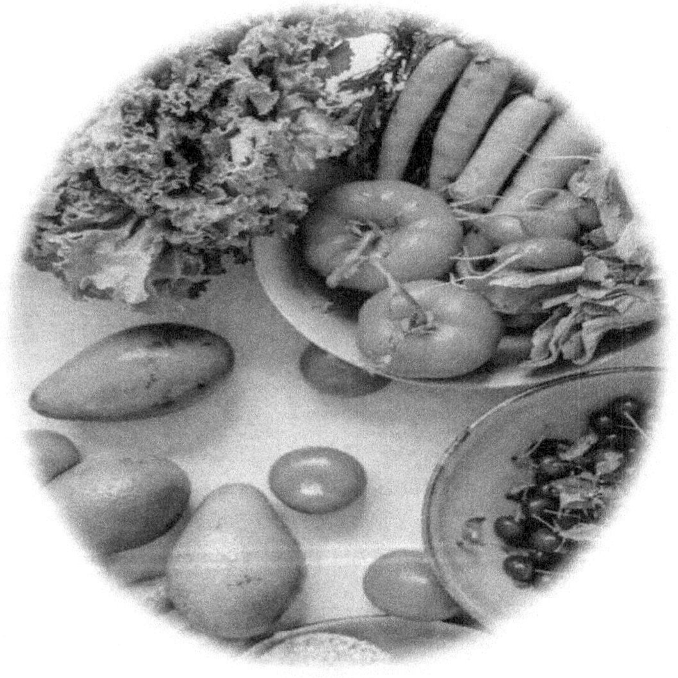

CHAPTER 15

Revitalize Your Body with Nourishing Detox Recipes

Toxins from various sources like air and water pollution, everyday products laden with chemicals, food additives, and even cigarette smoke can accumulate within our bodies.

These toxins, if not effectively removed by our natural biological processes, can lead to undesirable effects such as premature aging, bloating, and even weight gain.

Enter detoxification, or detox for short - the process of purging these toxic substances from our bodies. Detox diets have emerged as a simple and wholesome means to embark on this journey towards revitalized health.

Here's a breakdown of what to do and what to avoid in the world of detox diets:

The DOs: More Fiber and Water

A robust detox diet encourages the consumption of foods rich in fiber and ample hydration. Fiber aids in digestion and toxin removal, while water flushes out impurities from your system.

The DON'Ts: Caffeine, Carbonated Beverages, Sugars (Alcohol, Chocolate, and Yeast)

On the flip side, detox diets eschew caffeine, carbonated drinks, and sugars (yes, that includes alcohol, chocolate, and yeast), which can hamper the detox process.

For a more intensive detox, you might consider Dr. Kiki Sidhwa's recommendation: fasting for three days followed by consuming a single type of fruit per meal.

For instance, breakfast could consist of apples, lunch oranges or pineapples, and dinner a variety like grapes or bananas.

You're encouraged to eat as much of the chosen fruit as you desire during each meal, with non-sweetened fruit juice as an optional snack.

The key here is to stick to one fruit type per meal.

If this rigorous approach seems a bit much, detox diet recipes are here to help. These recipes are thoughtfully designed to provide essential nutrients and antioxidants for effective toxin elimination. Starting your detox diet by increasing fluid intake is a great first step.

Ginger Healing Tea with Turmeric

A delightful and efficacious addition to your detox diet, this tea combines ginger's cancer-fighting antioxidants with its abilities to alleviate nausea, motion sickness, and morning sickness.

To prepare, bring two cups of water to a boil, then add half a teaspoon of powdered ginger and half a teaspoon of turmeric. Simmer for ten minutes, strain into a mug, and add one tablespoon of maple syrup along with a dash of lemon extract.

Vegetable Super-Juice

Kickstart your detox diet mornings with this invigorating super-juice. It provides an energy boost, jumpstarts your digestive system, and keeps you going until lunch.

Blend a whole cucumber, four celery sticks, about an ounce of fresh spinach, and eight lettuce leaves with equal parts distilled water to aid the process.

A splash of lemon juice adds a zesty twist. Despite cucumbers being less nutritious than most fruits, their seeds offer vitamins A, B6, C, and K, potassium, thiamin, folate, and more.

Detox Diet Soup

For lunch, savor a high-energy detox diet soup. Blend one avocado with two spring onions, half a red or green pepper, a cucumber, half an ounce of fresh spinach, half a clove of garlic, and about one-third cup of yeast-free vegetable bouillon.

Squeeze in the juice of one lemon or lime, and if desired, season with coriander, cumin, or parsley. Blend until creamy, and voila - a nutritious soup to keep you fueled.

Warm Broccoli Soup

Come dinnertime, indulge in a comforting bowl of warm broccoli soup. Start by lightly steaming six to eight broccoli heads (about 5-6 minutes). Blend these steamed florets with half an avocado, one-third of a red onion, a celery stick, a handful of raw spinach, and an inch of ginger root.

Blend to your desired consistency, then season with cumin, Bragg liquid aminos, garlic, and ground black pepper to taste. This heartwarming favorite helps restore your body's chemical balance to its naturally alkaline state.

These are just a glimpse of the detox diet recipes readily available online. The key takeaway from this journey is to stay hydrated, nourish your body with essential nutrients, and avoid harmful additives, preservatives, and excessive sugars commonly found in modern processed foods.

Don't delay; embark on your journey to a healthier life with the transformative power of a detox diet.

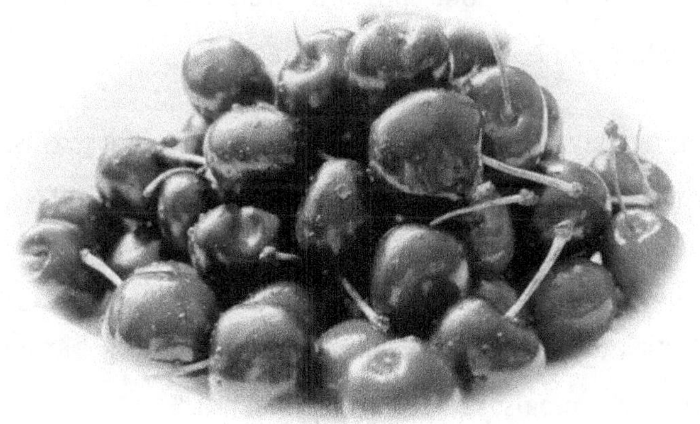

CHAPTER 16

Your Personal Roadmap to Weight Loss through Home Detox

In a world increasingly obsessed with weight and physique, most of us harbor the notion that shedding a few pounds could do us some good.

The journey to weight loss, as we all know, can be an exasperating one. Why? Because most conventional diets fail to address the root causes of weight gain - entrenched bad habits and compromised health.

From the day we're born, our bodies accumulate toxins, and in today's world, the assault of these toxins is relentless.

Fast food, processed meals, and our environment laden with air and water pollutants, not to mention a barrage of modern chemicals, create a toxic cocktail.

Genetic engineering of foods further complicates the puzzle of health.

However, the main culprit is our diet. Our bodies are inherently equipped to eliminate toxins and maintain equilibrium in temperature, pH levels, and biological functions.

There are three primary routes our bodies naturally employ for detoxification: adopting a more alkaline diet, restoring internal health equilibrium through biological processes, and expelling toxins via the digestive system.

When we consume excessively acidic diets, these natural processes become overburdened, leading to symptoms like fatigue, muscle pain, weight gain, and potentially severe ailments such as cancer.

If you're grappling with these symptoms or generally feeling subpar, it might be time for a home detox. Many experts and healthcare professionals deem home body detox a practical and logical solution for restoring a healthy chemical balance within the body.

An effective detox regimen can help you shed pounds, rekindle your energy, alleviate asthma and diabetes symptoms, and even slow down the aging process. Home body detox, unlike many popular diets, prioritizes your health before weight loss.

It might also prove to be a cost-effective alternative to the myriad diet programs vying for your attention today. As you work on your weight loss journey, the home body detox program simultaneously rejuvenates your body's innate cleansing abilities, steering it back toward a state of equilibrium.

Executing your home body detox program is convenient, primarily revolving around dietary choices and personal routines. You can detoxify your body sans specialized prescriptions or medications.

However, you might consider adding alkalizing water or vitamin/mineral supplements to expedite the detox process. An efficient home body detox program can be completed in as little as two to three weeks.

The core objectives of a home body detox program are weight loss, enhanced circulation, increased toxin elimination, colon cleansing, and nourishing the liver. The liver plays a pivotal role in natural detoxification, making its welfare a top priority.

Individuals who have embarked on home body detox programs often report faster weight loss compared to other diets and weight loss products. They also notice improvements such as clearer skin, better digestion, increased vitality, and regular bowel movements.

By adopting home body detox practices, you'll discover the foods that bolster your health. Fresh fruits and vegetables are the cornerstones, both for weight loss and restoring a healthy, alkaline pH level.

Say goodbye to processed meals, canned goods, meat- and dairy-centric dishes, and alcohol. Instead, welcome low-sugar fruits, leafy greens, alkaline water, virgin oils, stone-ground whole wheat products, lemon-infused water, and non-caffeinated, non-carbonated beverages.

Furthermore, increase your water intake significantly - experts recommend a minimum of four quarts daily during a detox program. Even after detox, aim to consume at least two quarts of water daily. Incorporating short one- or two-day fasts can accelerate the detoxification process.

One compelling reason to embark on a home body detox program is the acquisition of lifelong healthy habits that extend well beyond the weight loss phase.

It's crucial to understand that reverting to old eating habits will cause your body to reaccumulate toxins, leading to undesirable symptoms and weight gain. A consistent, balanced diet enables your body to naturally and effectively process and eliminate toxins, eliminating the need for supplements or medications.

The choice is yours - opt for a healthy life and embrace positive lifestyle changes, or succumb to an unhealthy existence with poor choices, which could eventually lead you back to contemplating a home body detox program.

Remember, there's no need to rush into these changes all at once. You can gradually modify your dietary habits, initiating some alterations now and integrating others progressively. Begin incorporating more regular physical activity into your life, starting with short walks and gradually building up to a more intensive exercise regimen. Don't forget to detox your mind; allocate time daily to nurture your psychological and emotional well-being, mitigating stressors that contribute to ill health.

Lastly, a crucial piece of advice - before embarking on any diet or home body detox program, consult your physician to rule out any underlying medical conditions that require medical treatment before initiating detox.

Your doctor might also provide additional insights to enhance your detox experience and guide you towards a new, healthy, and joyful lifestyle.

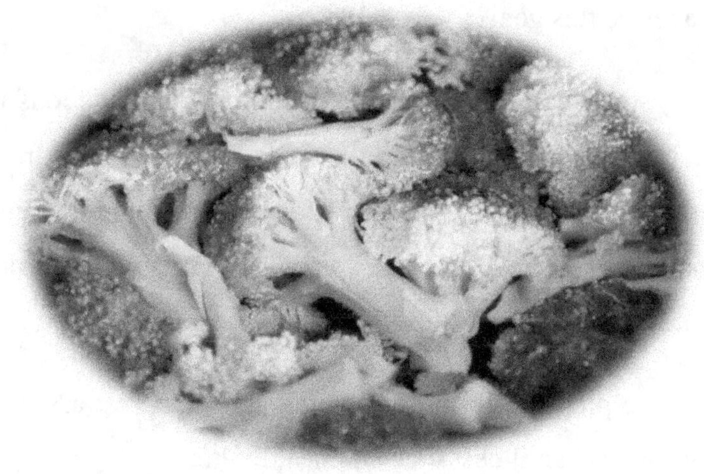

CHAPTER 17

7 Days to a Toxin-Free You: The Power of Internal Cleansing

Understanding the root causes of diseases and illnesses is paramount to steering clear of them. As medical expenses continue to soar, falling ill becomes an increasingly costly affair. This reality drives people to prioritize their health. But are individuals ready to make necessary compromises to achieve this goal?

Well, staying healthy entails consuming the right foods in the right quantities at the right times and abstaining from detrimental habits like excessive alcohol consumption and smoking. Achieving and maintaining good health necessitates a shift in lifestyle as much as possible.

If you're prepared to make these adjustments, rest assured, you can lead an illness-free and healthy life.

Years of consuming various beverages and food items, combined with environmental factors, render your body susceptible to a myriad of diseases and illnesses.

Toxins accumulate when the body's natural detoxification processes become overwhelmed by the toxic load. This accumulation of toxins can lead to a host of health problems and ultimately result in sickness.

The detox diet, featuring natural herbs and supplements, is gaining widespread recognition. These foods facilitate the elimination of toxins through the body's organs, including the liver, lungs, skin, kidneys, and intestines. Additionally, the body's lymphatic system plays a crucial role in removing toxins.

Nevertheless, it's imperative to consult with your physician before embarking on any detox diet program, as only a healthcare professional can assess your current health status and provide guidance on whether your chosen path is safe.

If you are already experiencing a toxic buildup, specific symptoms may indicate this condition. Furthermore, when you commence your detox regimen, these symptoms may initially intensify.

However, it's crucial to remain patient, as this phase signifies that your body is undergoing detoxification.

For those seeking an efficient method to eliminate toxins from their bodies, a detox body cleanser is a valuable option. This cleanser has been proven to cleanse the body's internal organs in just seven days.

By utilizing a body cleanser, you can initiate a seven-day detox program to eliminate unwanted toxins from your body.

These detox body cleansers are available in various forms, such as fiber packets or tablets, and are composed of natural herbs and fibers.

Within a week, you'll likely experience a noticeable surge in energy, revitalization, and detoxification. Some individuals have even reported experiencing effects after just one day.

Although detox body cleansers are generally affordable, their price should not be the sole consideration when prioritizing a healthy body. These cleansers are user-friendly and, despite their herbal composition, are palatable and easy to digest. Their primary objective is to comprehensively cleanse your body, and they excel at doing just that.

Detox body cleansers are readily available at leading drugstores and online retailers. If you're looking for rapid results in your quest for a toxin-free body, consider embarking on a seven-day body cleansing journey. Your revitalized, detoxified self will thank you.

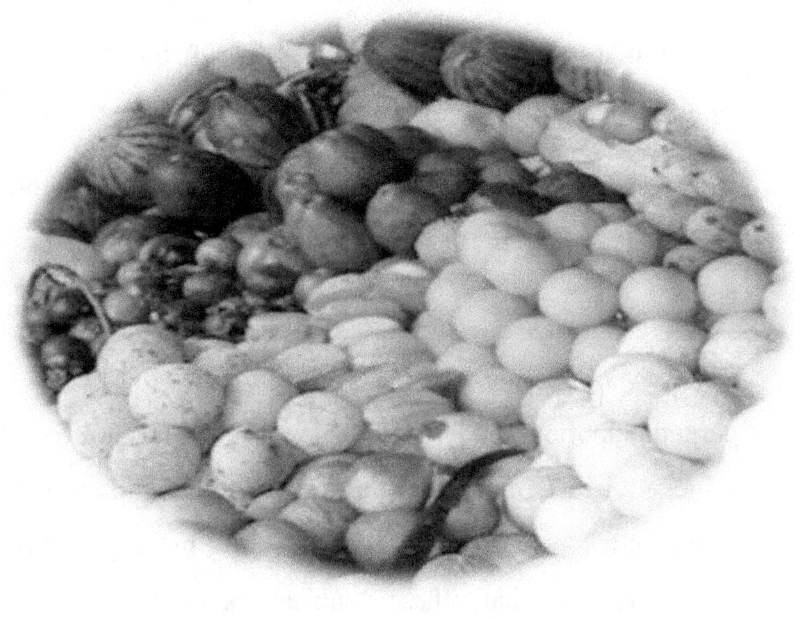

CHAPTER 18

The Natural Path to Detox

Have you ever experienced moments when your body feels inexplicably heavy, your energy levels plummet, and even the thought of moving seems like an insurmountable task? You might resort to excessive eating or lighting up a cigarette, hoping for a quick boost of vitality.

However, these habits only provide fleeting relief while silently fostering the accumulation of toxins within your body.

In our ever-evolving world, we aspire to keep our bodies in perpetual motion, ready for action at a moment's notice. To achieve this, we often turn to artificial body stimulants such as cigarettes, coffee, drugs, diet pills, and more, under the misconception that these substances will keep us consistently active.

Sadly, these stimulants tend to sap our energy and give rise to a host of emotional ailments like depression, sickness, and headaches. Additionally, they leave behind a trail of toxins in their wake.

But what exactly are toxins? Toxins are substances that pose harm to the body, generally categorized into two types: internal or endogenous toxins and external or exogenous toxins.

External toxins originate from sources outside the body, such as tobacco smoke, car exhaust, industrial pollution, and drugs.

Conversely, internal toxins result from bacterial or viral infections, while the body also generates its own toxins, known as autogenous toxins, as part of the metabolic process.

The body naturally rids itself of these harmful substances through a vital process called detoxification.

Detoxification is the body's mechanism for expelling accumulated toxic compounds found in the bloodstream, liver, kidneys, and bowels, as well as those lurking within body fat. The most straightforward approach to eliminating toxins is through a body detox regimen centered on a natural diet, with an emphasis on vegetables and fruits.

For those leading bustling lives, it's high time to replace artificial stimulants with natural alternatives to regain energy and vitality.

The most commonly used stimulants include cigarettes, red meat, diet pills, coffee, and refined sugar.

Sugar is renowned for its quick energy surge, often found in carbonated drinks. Yet, refined white sugar poses severe risks to the body.

Cola and ketchup contain substantial amounts of refined white sugar, which can be swapped for healthier alternatives like brown sugars and cane sugars. Fruit juices offer a similar energy boost without the detrimental effects.

Late-night workers frequently rely on coffee to stay awake. A healthier alternative is Chinese or Japanese green tea, which contains caffeine for alertness without the stomach irritation. Some individuals turn to diet pills to replace meals, a common practice among athletes, especially during competitions due to their energy-boosting properties. Despite being aware of the side effects, these athletes persist. Instead, they should embrace the natural detoxifying abilities of fruits.

Cigarette smokers often believe that smoking enhances cognitive function, but in reality, it primarily leads to cancer. Carrots can provide a similar mental uplift, but in a much healthier and beneficial manner.

This is why we've been encouraged to consume vegetables and fruits from a young age. These foods are celebrated for their ability to promote a healthy body, enabling it to combat and expel toxins effectively.

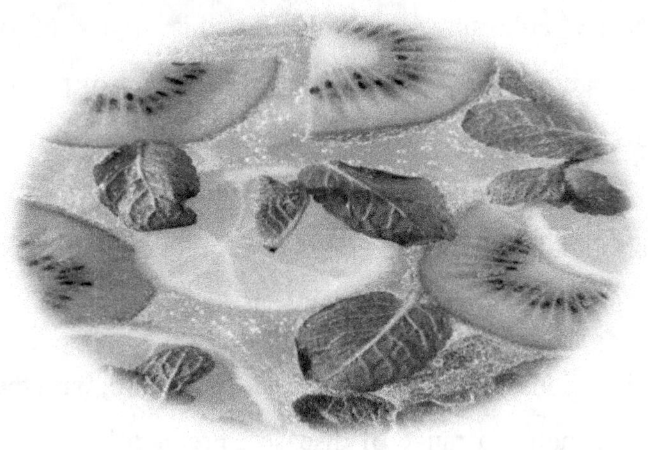

CHAPTER 19

The Imperative of Detoxification in Our Modern World

In our contemporary society, the issue of toxicity has risen to alarming levels, demanding our immediate attention. The fast-paced, modern lifestyle has unwittingly become a breeding ground for toxins to accumulate within the human body.

The primary culprits responsible for this toxic influx include air and water pollution, the proliferation of potent chemicals, radiation exposure, and nuclear power generation. On top of this, we're ingesting a slew of new chemicals and drugs, often coupled with an overindulgence in sugar, processed foods, stimulants, and sedatives.

The ramifications of this toxic overload are severe, with the potential to induce a range of diseases. Frequently, cancer and various cardiovascular ailments can be traced back to elevated toxin levels in the body. Allergies, obesity, skin disorders, arthritis, and a host of other health issues are also frequently linked to this accumulation.

Moreover, toxin build-up manifests as constant headaches, persistent fatigue, gastrointestinal distress, bodily discomfort, and even chronic coughs, all of which contribute to a weakened immune system.

Detoxification, or the process of cleansing the body, emerges as a vital solution to mitigate both acute and chronic illnesses resulting from toxin exposure. This transformative process entails the removal of harmful chemicals and toxins present within the body.

Detox programs can be tailored to suit individual needs, varying in duration from short-term to long-term interventions. These programs are especially effective for those grappling with addiction, as they help individuals break free from harmful habits.

Toxicity operates on two fronts: external and internal. External toxicity stems from environmental exposure, which can occur through inhalation, physical contact, or ingestion of toxins. Additionally, external toxicity encompasses the chemicals found in the foods we consume. Many drugs, allergens, and food additives introduce toxic elements into the body.

It's worth noting that even nutrients, sodium, and water contain a certain degree of toxicity. In contrast, internally produced toxins arise from the body's daily, routine functions.

Biochemical and cellular activities generate substances that necessitate elimination. These substances, commonly referred to as free radicals or biochemical toxins, have the potential to incite cellular and tissue irritation, disrupting the normal functioning of bodily cells or organs.

Furthermore, various foreign invaders, such as bacteria, parasites, intestinal bacteria, yeasts, and microbes, produce metabolic byproducts that contribute to internal toxins. Interestingly, our thoughts, stress, and emotions can also instigate the generation of biochemical toxins.

In essence, nearly everyone must engage in some form of detoxification to maintain optimal bodily function. Cleansing and detoxification constitute the third facet of nutritional action. Although individuals who maintain a balanced diet and avoid excesses necessitate less intensive detoxification, those who consume diets rich in refined foods, high fats, dairy products, and medications produce a substantial toxin load, compelling a need for detoxification.

Fasting serves as another detox therapy embraced by many. It stands as one of the oldest and most comprehensive natural human treatments.

During detoxification, dead cells and waste are systematically cleared from the body, reinvigorating its natural processes and rekindling its innate healing potential. Countless individuals attest to the remarkable results of a well-structured cleansing program.

Detoxifying the body is pivotal to maintaining good health. While our bodies possess the capacity to handle a certain level of toxic content, it's prudent to keep these levels to a minimum by adjusting our dietary choices.

The transformative power of detoxification is undeniable, promising a bolstered immune system and a healthier body. By taking these steps, you can potentially avert numerous diseases and lead a more vibrant and fulfilling life.

CHAPTER 20

The Holistic Approach to Detoxifying Mind, Body, and Spirit

Spirituality has woven itself into the fabric of many lives. For believers, it's a guiding force, influencing our choices and actions. Today, the pursuit of holistic living is surging in popularity. This lifestyle advocates not just physical health, but a profound sense of spiritual well-being.

Devotees of spirituality often proclaim that physical health is incomplete without spiritual vitality. In this intricate dance of existence, the body, mind, and spirit are inextricably linked. Achieving true purification requires harmony among these elements.

Regrettably, amid the hustle and bustle of contemporary life, our spiritual selves often receive scant attention. We find ourselves caught up in paying bills, meeting deadlines, amassing wealth, socializing, and striving to maintain physical well-being.

While these pursuits are valid, they occasionally overshadow our spiritual needs. Yet, if the aim is to cleanse our entire being, a holistic detox encompassing mind, body, and soul emerges as a potent solution.

The human body possesses its own mechanisms for detoxification, but at times, the toxic burden becomes overwhelming. This is where detox products step in to aid the body's natural processes.

These products facilitate detoxification, infusing fresh vitality and energy. Improved bowel function and healthier skin often accompany a body detox, amplifying its benefits.

Mental detoxification is another facet of this comprehensive approach. The mind, like the body, needs cleansing.

Eradicating negative thoughts and fostering positivity are central to this process. In Eastern cultures, the practice of psychoneuroimmunology, dating back centuries, attests to the profound connection between the mind and body.

This method encourages patients to focus on their thoughts, visualizing healing energy coursing through the organs requiring rejuvenation. Successful implementation of this technique accelerates the healing process, underscoring the profound mind-body connection.

Visualization is the linchpin here, but for effective mind detox, professional guidance is often invaluable. Multiple techniques are available, each tailored to individual needs.

Spiritual well-being constitutes a vital aspect of life deserving of attention. Prayer, the most universally recognized expression of spirituality, transcends cultural and religious boundaries.

Prayer is deeply personal, with no universally prescribed form. It can be practiced anywhere, in any manner, as long as it emanates from the heart, grounded in faith. The key is finding a method of prayer that resonates with your spirit, setting the stage for spiritual detoxification.

These strategies represent just a glimpse into the multifaceted world of holistic detoxification for mind, body, and spirit. If you desire a comprehensive approach and wish to ensure your journey is harmonious and effective, consider seeking guidance from experienced professionals who can tailor a program to your unique needs.

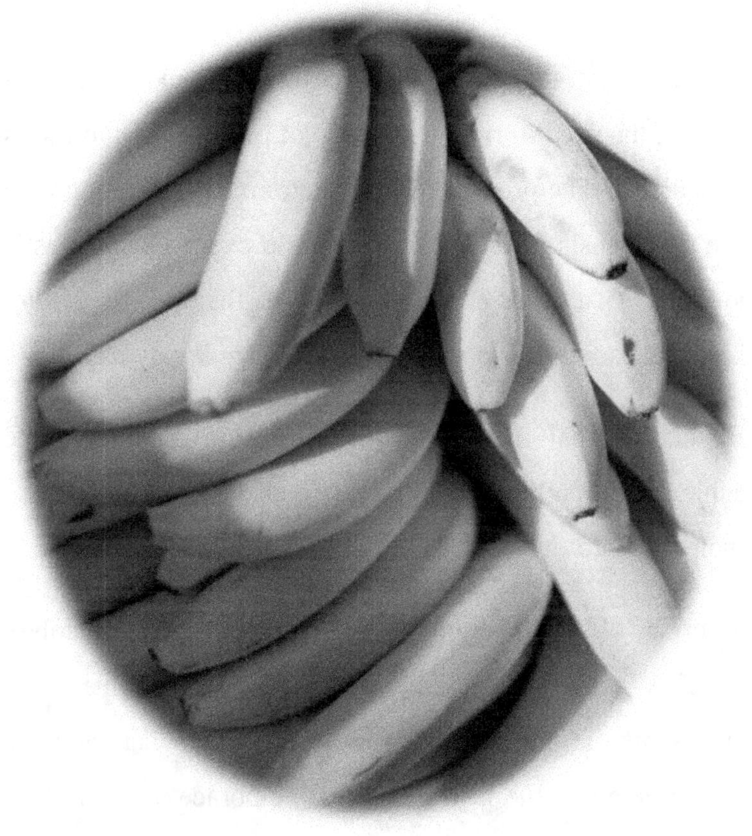

CHAPTER 21

Revitalize Your Body with Natural Herbs for Detox

In our quest for optimal body function and boundless energy, the need to rid our systems of accumulated toxins is undeniable. The process of body detoxification through the use of cleansing herbs is not a single event but a holistic journey. It's a series of steps, a lifestyle that aids the body's innate capacity to expel toxins efficiently, day by day.

Beyond herbal remedies, detoxification can also be achieved by curbing the intake of various toxins that find their way into our bodies.

Steering clear of culprits like refined sugar, alcohol, caffeine, pharmaceuticals, tobacco, household chemicals, and synthetic or petroleum-based products serves as a potent detox method. In their stead, embrace a diet rich in natural, organic foods, incorporate regular exercise, and maintain proper hydration. Gradual changes often prove more manageable for the body compared to abrupt detox procedures.

Let's delve into some remarkable herbs renowned for their detoxifying properties:

Milk Thistle and Dandelion Root: Milk thistle strengthens and cleanses the liver, safeguarding it and promoting regeneration through silymarin. Meanwhile, dandelion root aids in purging waste from the kidneys and gall bladder.

Psyllium Husks and Seeds: Rich in fiber, these gems gently act as natural laxatives. Soaking the seeds in water is a common practice, and psyllium is celebrated as an adaptogen, supporting healthy bowel functions. It's also beneficial for managing conditions like diarrhea. After soaking, its gelatinous texture effectively absorbs toxins, making it a prime choice for body detox.

Gravel Root (Joe Pye Weed) and Hydrangea Root: These herbs play a crucial role in dissolving, expelling, and preventing kidney and bladder stones and crystals.

Ensuring unobstructed kidney function is vital for toxin elimination.

Nettle: Not just for the urinary system, nettle possesses detoxifying properties that extend further. Yet, similar to juniper berries, excessive use can yield similar effects.

Cascara Sagrada: Another natural laxative, it aids in strengthening the colon muscles and is considered safe for prolonged use.

Essential Oils: Cypress, celery, basil, lemon, rosemary, fennel, patchouli, and thyme oils play a pivotal role in flushing out toxins nestled beneath the skin. They also stimulate lymphatic circulation.

Alder Buckthorn's Bark: Although highly effective, it should be dried and stored for at least a year before use, as fresh bark can be overly potent and potentially toxic.

Juniper Berries: Promoting overall urinary system health, juniper berries fortify and detoxify the kidneys, bladder, and urinary tract. However, extended use may burden the kidneys, so moderation is key.

Burdock Roots and Seeds: These herbs share qualities with nettle but are more potent. They act as a cleansing, mild diuretic and can even help remove heavy metals from the body.

Embarking on a home-based body detox journey opens doors to various natural remedies, harnessing the incredible potential of these herbs. Rediscover the joy of rejuvenation as you pamper your body, and revel in the newfound vitality coursing through your veins.

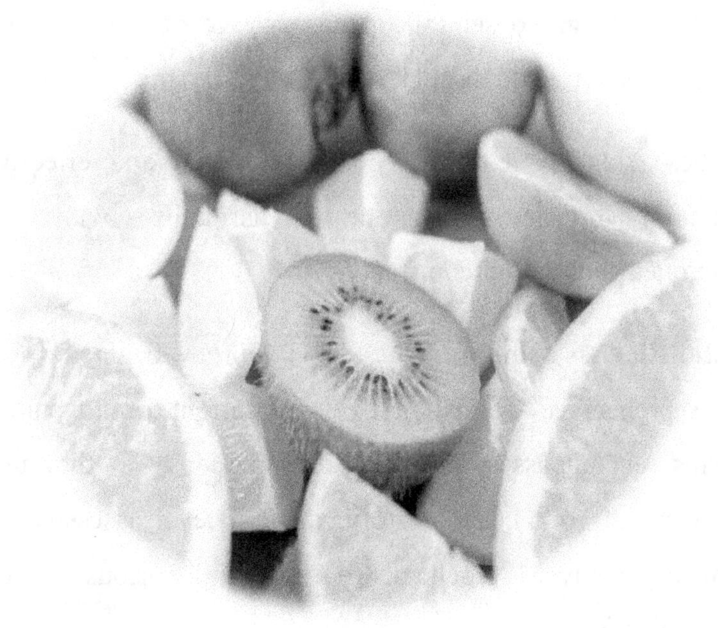

CHAPTER 22

Your Guide to Natural Body Detox

Embarking on a detox or cleansing program may seem daunting, but fear not, for it's a transformative journey worth taking. To set sail on this voyage of renewal, you must first navigate through several essential procedures.

These steps pave the way for a tailored and effective natural body detox plan, one that harmonizes with your unique needs and circumstances.

Holistic Assessment: Your detox journey begins with a comprehensive evaluation of your current health status. This encompasses physical examinations, a thorough review of your health history, mineral level assessments, dietary analysis, biochemistry tests, and various related examinations.

These tests serve as navigational charts, plotting the course for your body's cleansing voyage.

They unveil crucial insights into your health, helping to determine the most suitable natural procedures for your detoxification.

Customized Detox Plan: Armed with the insights from your health assessment, your detox plan takes shape. It's a blueprint meticulously crafted to align with your individual health requirements, lifestyle, genetic predispositions, and dietary choices.

Remember, there's no one-size-fits-all solution in detoxification. Your plan is a personalized map to wellness.

The Power of Nutrition: Proper nourishment is your vessel for a successful detox journey. Individuals facing nutrient deficiencies, fatigue, or organ underperformance will require a diet rich in essential nutrients and proteins.

This dietary foundation helps to rejuvenate your system. In some cases, short-term fasting, light eating, and fruit or vegetable juice consumption can serve as a powerful tool for eliminating accumulated waste and preparing your body for a healthier future.

Harnessing Nature's Herbs: Various organs in your body tend to accumulate toxins over time, especially the colon and liver. Specific detox programs target these areas for revitalization.

Fiber supplements, including acidophilus culture, aloe vera powder, and bentonite clay, support colon cleansing and toning. Enemas with diluted coffee, herbal blends, and water aid in liver detoxification.

The Dance of Exercise: Exercise is a spirited partner in your detox expedition. It prompts sweat, expelling toxins through the skin, boosts metabolism, and overall aids in detoxification.

Regular aerobic workouts maintain your body's toxin-free rhythm. Remember, moderation is key; excessive exercise may elevate toxic production, so balance is essential.

The Art of Cleansing: Regular cleansing rituals, including bathing and dry skin brushing, are pivotal for toxin elimination. They refresh your skin, a vital excretory organ, and invigorate your entire system.

The Magic of Massage: Massage therapy holds a special place in detox programs. It not only supports body elimination functions but also induces relaxation, melting away tension and mental stress. It's a vital element in your rejuvenation journey.

Tranquility and Recharge: Amid detoxification, moments of rest, relaxation, and renewal are paramount. Your body and mind crave these breaks to recalibrate. Practices like yoga offer the dual benefits of enhancing your breath control and cultivating an active, balanced aura.

As you navigate these natural procedures, remember that the path to cleansing your body is your own. Choose the procedures that resonate with your unique needs and preferences. A detoxified body is a healthier and happier vessel for your life's adventures.

Conclusion

The journey to an effortless body detox is a path towards renewed vitality and wellness with ease. This process is not about drastic measures or extreme sacrifices; instead, it's a gentle and sustainable way to reset your body, mind, and spirit.

By adopting holistic practices such as mindful nutrition, regular exercise, and relaxation techniques, you can gradually remove toxins, boost your energy levels, and enhance your overall well-being.

Remember, the key lies in consistency and balance. As you make these positive changes a part of your daily life, you'll discover that revitalizing your health can be a natural and enjoyable process.

So, embark on this journey with confidence, knowing that with each small effort, you are renewing your vitality and embracing a life of lasting wellness.